Also by Andrew D Beattie

All About
All About Crohn's Disease

A - Z
A - Z of Mental Health

Inside The Mind
Complex ADHD

Mental Health
Breaking Through Executive Dysfunction: Strategies for
Patients with Complex Trauma and ADHD
Anxiety Disorders Unmasked - Tackling Procrastination Head
On
INSIDE THE MIND - Exploring Anxiety Disorders
Personality Traits Explained

Standalone
My Naked Soul

Table of Contents

INSIDE THE MIND:

Complex ADHD

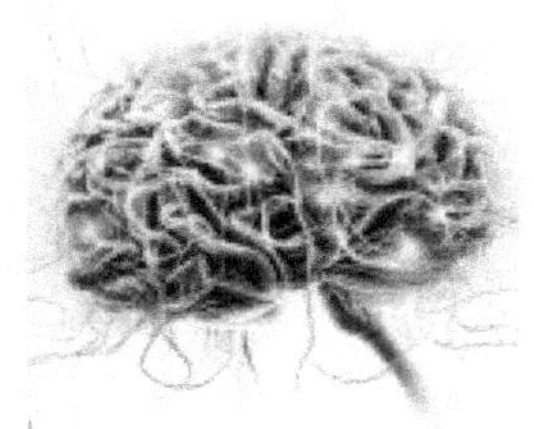

Andrew D Beattie

INSIDE THE MIND:

Complex ADHD

Written by

Andrew D Beattie

2023

COMPLEX ADHD

Chapter 1: Introduction to Complex ADHD

Definition of Complex ADHD: Is it Real?

Imagine a symphony orchestra, where each musician is an expert in their own instrument. However, for the orchestra to create harmonious music, all the musicians must play in sync. Now, consider the human brain as this orchestra, with different parts performing different functions. In a person with Attention-Deficit/Hyperactivity Disorder (ADHD), it's as if some musicians are out of sync, disrupting the harmony.

ADHD is a neurodevelopmental disorder characterized by persistent patterns of inattention, impulsivity, and hyperactivity. People with ADHD may have trouble focusing, controlling impulsive behaviours, or be overly active. It's like the drummer playing too fast or the flutist playing too slow.

Now, imagine if some musicians were not just out of sync but also playing a completely different song. This is what happens in Complex ADHD.

Complex ADHD is not a separate disorder, but a term used to describe ADHD accompanied by one or more additional mental health conditions. These can include mood disorders like depression or bipolar disorder, anxiety disorders, obsessive-compulsive disorder (OCD), substance use disorders, and others. The presence of these additional conditions can complicate the diagnosis, treatment, and management of ADHD.

For instance, symptoms of the comorbid condition may overlap with those of ADHD, making it challenging to distinguish between the two. The flutist might be playing slow because they're part of a melancholic melody (depression) or because they can't keep up with the rhythm (ADHD). Additionally, these comorbid conditions can exacerbate the symptoms of ADHD or

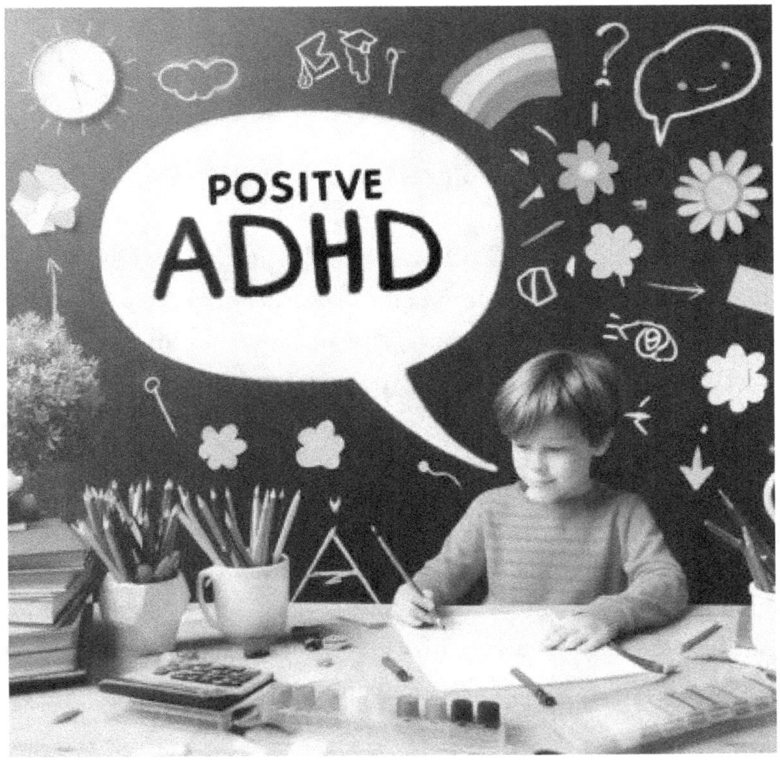

vice versa. The melancholic melody might make the drummer lose his rhythm even more.

It's important to note that not everyone with ADHD has Complex ADHD. Some individuals may have ADHD without any other mental health conditions. However, research suggests that comorbidities are common in people with ADHD.

In conclusion, Complex ADHD is like an orchestra playing multiple songs at once. It's a multifaceted condition that requires a comprehensive approach to diagnosis and treatment. It underscores the importance of considering the whole person and all the music they're playing, not just their ADHD symptoms, to provide the most effective care.

The prevalence of Complex ADHD

ADHD, OR ATTENTION-Deficit/Hyperactivity Disorder, is a common neurodevelopmental disorder that affects both children and adults. It's characterized by persistent patterns of inattention, impulsivity, and hyperactivity. In the United States alone, it's estimated that over 9 percent of children aged 2 to 17 years old will be diagnosed with ADHD at some point in their lives. That's a staggering 6.1 million children!

However, ADHD is not confined to the United States. It's a global concern affecting people from all walks of life. Worldwide, the prevalence of ADHD in children is estimated to be between 5.29% and 7.2%, and around 2.5% in adults.

In the United Kingdom, it's estimated that between 3% to 4% of adults have ADHD. This means that in a room of 100 adults, there could be up to 4 individuals living with ADHD.

In Scotland, the prevalence rates for ADHD are about 5% of school age children. This means that in a typical classroom of 20 students, there could be at least one child with ADHD.

Now, let's talk about Complex ADHD. This term refers to individuals who have been diagnosed with ADHD and also have one or more additional mental health conditions. These can include mood disorders like depression or bipolar disorder, anxiety disorders, obsessive-compulsive disorder (OCD), substance use disorders, and others.

Research suggests that as many as 80% of adults with ADHD have at least one co-existing psychiatric disorder, while approximately 60% of children with ADHD have at least one co-occurring condition. This means that out of the millions of individuals diagnosed with ADHD worldwide, a significant proportion also live with additional mental health conditions.

These statistics underscore the complexity and prevalence of Complex ADHD. It's a condition that affects millions of individuals worldwide and requires comprehensive care and understanding from healthcare providers, educators, parents, and society as a whole.

Chapter 2: The Causes of Complex ADHD

The types of events and factors that can cause Complex ADHD

Complex ADHD, also known as ADHD with comorbidities, is a term used to describe a diagnosis of ADHD along with one or more additional mental health conditions. The exact cause of ADHD isn't fully understood, but it's believed to be a combination of several factors:

Genetic Factors

ADHD tends to run in families, and, in most cases, it's thought the genes you inherit from your parents are a significant factor in developing the condition[1]. Research shows that parents and siblings of someone with ADHD are more likely to have ADHD themselves[1]. However, the way ADHD is inherited is likely to be complex and is not thought to be related to a single genetic fault[1].

Brain Function and Structure

Research has identified a number of possible differences in the brains of people with ADHD from those without the condition[1]. For example, studies involving brain scans have suggested that certain areas of the brain may be smaller in people with ADHD, whereas other areas may be larger[1]. Other studies have suggested that people with ADHD may have an imbalance in the level of neurotransmitters in the brain, or that these chemicals may not work properly

Environmental Factors

Certain environmental factors such as exposure to lead as a child, low birth weight, maternal smoking during pregnancy, and alcohol exposure during pregnancy are associated with ADHD. Other risk factors include preterm delivery, epilepsy, acquired brain injury, lead exposure, iron deficiency, psychosocial adversity, and adverse maternal mental health.

In terms of Complex ADHD specifically, the additional mental health conditions that co-occur with ADHD can also be influenced by a combination of genetic, environmental, and psychological factors. These can include mood disorders (such as depression or bipolar disorder), anxiety disorders, obsessive-compulsive disorder (OCD), substance use disorders, and others.

It's important to note that these factors do not cause ADHD or Complex ADHD directly but rather increase the risk of developing these conditions. The exact interplay between these factors is still a subject of ongoing research.

Chapter 3: Symptoms of Complex ADHD

Symptoms similar to ADHD

Let's explore the symptoms similar to ADHD, which can sometimes lead to confusion or misdiagnosis:

Anxiety Disorders: About one-fifth of kids with ADHD also have some type of anxiety disorder, including separation anxiety, social anxiety, or general anxiety. Children with ADHD are more likely than others to experience anxiety. The type of medication they take for ADHD can make a big difference if they also have anxiety. Stimulants can make anxiety worse, but antidepressants can help with it.

Depression: Approximately 1 in 7 children with ADHD are also diagnosed with depression. Experts believe that stress from having ADHD could worsen depression. Additionally, certain ADHD medications have side effects that can mimic symptoms of depression, such as changes in eating and sleeping habits.

Autism Spectrum Disorder (ASD): Like ADHD, ASD affects brain development. These two conditions sometimes co-occur, although experts aren't entirely sure why. Both ASD and ADHD can cause children to hyperfocus on one thing. However, kids on the autism spectrum may avoid eye contact, be less interested in playing with other kids, and experience delayed speech development.

Oppositional Defiant Disorder (ODD): Children who frequently lose their temper, refuse to follow rules, argue with adults, and say mean things to others are often diagnosed with ODD. While some of this behaviour is "normal" for 2-3-year-olds, it becomes problematic if it persists as the child gets older. ODD is more common in boys than girls and usually improves within three years in about 60% of cases.

Remember that accurate diagnosis is essential because many conditions share symptoms with ADHD. If your child exhibits ADHD-like behaviours, consult a doctor to explore all possibilities before reaching a conclusion.

Additional symptoms unique to Complex ADHD

COMPLEX ADHD, ALSO known as ADHD with comorbidities, refers to a diagnosis of ADHD along with one or more additional mental health conditions. These additional conditions can lead to symptoms that are not typically associated with ADHD alone.

For instance, if a person with ADHD also has an anxiety disorder, they may experience symptoms such as excessive worry, restlessness, and difficulty concentrating due to worry. These symptoms are not typically associated with ADHD alone but can occur in individuals with Complex ADHD.

Similarly, if a person with ADHD also has a mood disorder such as depression, they may experience symptoms such as persistent feelings of sadness, loss of interest in previously enjoyed activities, and fatigue. Again, these are not symptoms of ADHD alone but can occur in individuals with Complex ADHD.

In addition to these psychological symptoms, individuals with Complex ADHD may also experience socio-occupational dysfunction. This can include difficulties in school or work performance, unemployment, unstable relationships, and poor physical and mental health3.

It's important to note that the presence of these additional symptoms can complicate the diagnosis and treatment of ADHD. For example, some symptoms of anxiety or depression can mimic or exacerbate symptoms of ADHD, making it more challenging to accurately diagnose and effectively treat the condition.

In conclusion, Complex ADHD is characterized by a range of symptoms that extend beyond those typically associated with ADHD. These additional symptoms reflect the presence of one or more co-occurring mental health conditions and underscore the complexity of this condition.

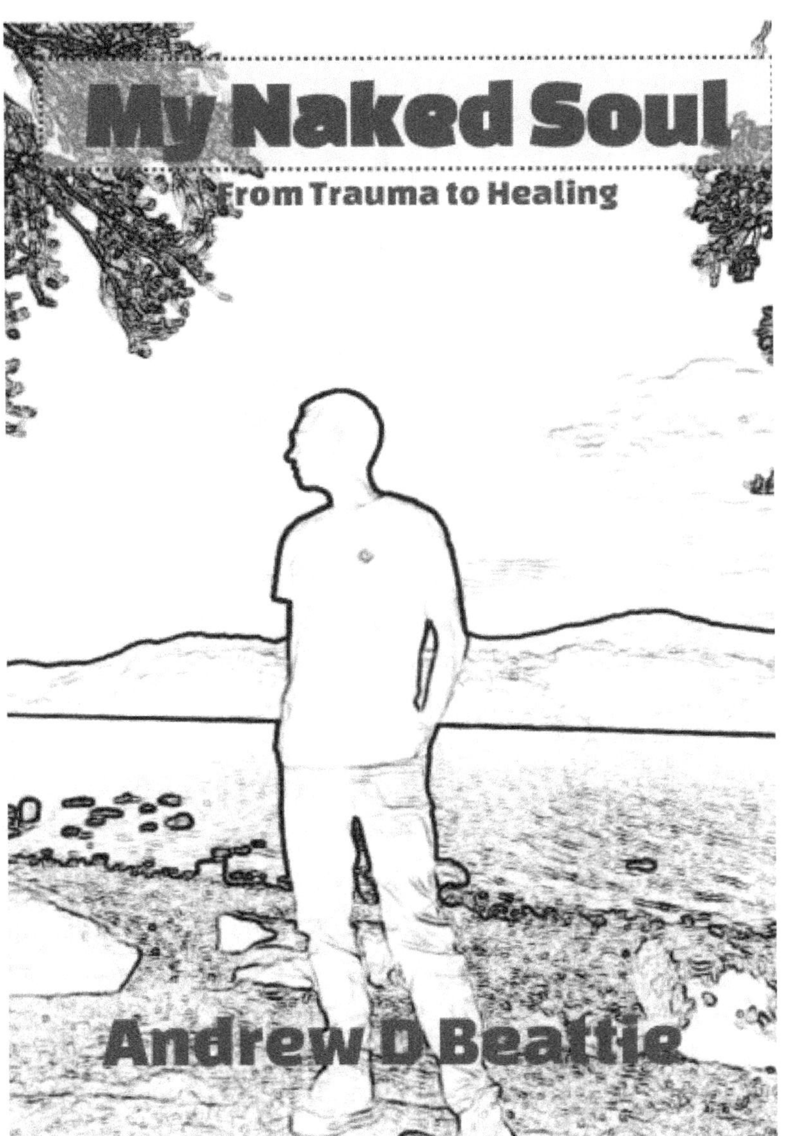
My Naked Soul
From Trauma to Healing
Andrew D Beattie

Chapter 4: The Impact of Complex ADHD

How Complex ADHD affects the brain and body

Let's delve deeper into how Complex ADHD affects the brain and body:

Neurological Differences: An ADHD brain isn't wired the same way as a non-ADHD brain. Specific differences in structure, function, and chemistry contribute to the condition. For instance:

Norepinephrine Levels: One significant difference is the level of norepinephrine, a neurotransmitter synthesized from dopamine. Lower levels of both dopamine and norepinephrine are linked to ADHD. This is because these neurotransmitters play a crucial role in regulating attention and activity levels. When their levels are low, it can lead to symptoms such as inattention, hyperactivity, and impulsivity.

Brain Regions: The structure of the ADHD brain differs in areas like the frontal cortex, which regulates behaviour and attention, and the limbic regions, influencing emotions and motivation. These areas are often smaller or less active in people with ADHD, which can lead to difficulties with impulse control, emotional regulation, and attention.

Default Mode Network (DMN): In ADHD, the DMN is more often activated, leading to constant distraction from tasks due to unrelated thoughts. The DMN is a network of brain regions that are active when the mind is at rest and not focused on the outside world. It's involved in introspective activities such as daydreaming or thinking about others' perspectives. In people with ADHD, the DMN may be overactive, leading to difficulties with attention and focus.

Brain Development: ADHD can change brain development. Physical changes in the brain lead to symptoms like decreased attention and increased hyperactivity. Research shows deficits in neural networks linked to attention and executive function in individuals with ADHD.

Body Impact: Beyond the brain, ADHD can also have physical effects on the body. People with ADHD often have high energy levels and may have difficulty sitting still. They may also have sleep problems, which can affect overall health and well-being.

When it comes to Complex ADHD specifically, the presence of additional mental health conditions can further impact both brain function and physical health. For example, if a person with Complex ADHD also has an anxiety disorder, they may experience physical symptoms such as restlessness or a rapid heart rate. Similarly, if they have a mood disorder such as depression, they may experience physical symptoms such as fatigue or changes in appetite.

In conclusion, Complex ADHD affects not only brain function but also physical health. Understanding these impacts is crucial for managing the condition effectively.

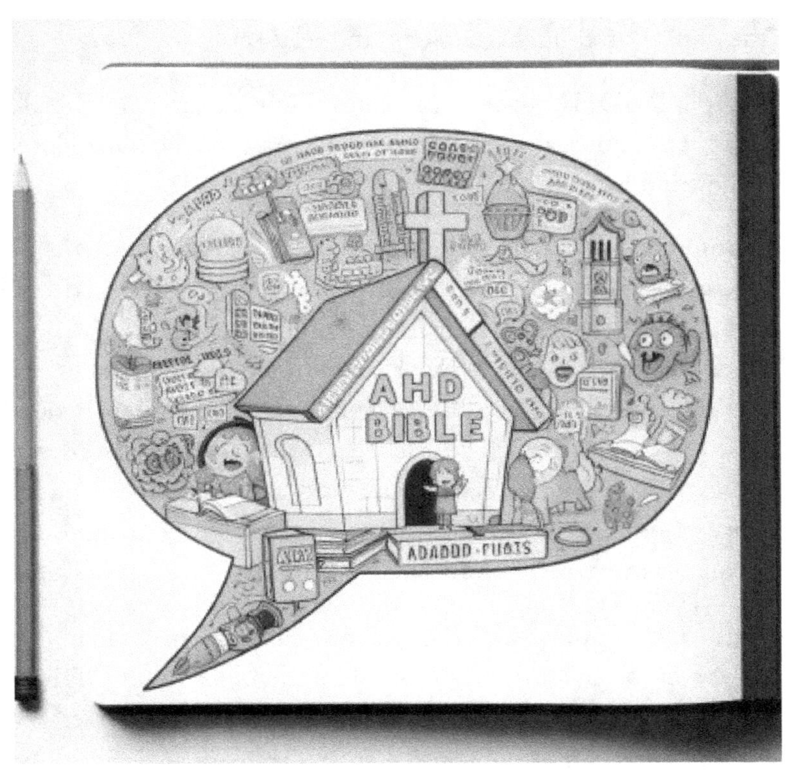
AHD
BIBLE
ADADDD · FUATS

The impact on thoughts, actions, and relationships

Complex ADHD can significantly impact an individual's thoughts, actions, and relationships. Here's a more detailed look at these impacts:

Thoughts: Individuals with Complex ADHD often experience intrusive thoughts that can be distressing and disruptive. These thoughts can be related to their ADHD symptoms (such as worries about forgetting things or not being able to focus) or to their co-occurring conditions (such as fears related to anxiety disorders or negative self-beliefs related to depressive disorders). These intrusive thoughts can lead to difficulties with concentration and decision-making and can contribute to feelings of overwhelm or distress.

Actions: Complex ADHD can also impact an individual's actions or behaviours. For example, individuals with ADHD often struggle with impulsivity, which can lead to hasty actions without considering the consequences. This impulsivity can be exacerbated by co-occurring conditions such as substance use disorders or oppositional defiant disorder. Additionally, individuals with Complex ADHD may struggle with consistent follow-through on tasks or commitments, which can impact various areas of life including work, school, and personal projects.

Relationships: The symptoms of Complex ADHD can also have a significant impact on relationships. The impulsivity and inconsistency associated with ADHD can lead to misunderstandings or conflicts with others. Additionally, co-occurring conditions such as anxiety disorders or depressive disorders can also impact relationships. For example, the social anxiety that often co-occurs with ADHD can lead to avoidance of social situations, while the irritability associated with depressive disorders can strain interpersonal interactions.

Self-Perception: Individuals with Complex ADHD often struggle with self-esteem and self-perception. They may internalize their struggles with ADHD as personal failures, leading to negative self-beliefs. These negative self-perceptions can be reinforced by the challenges they face due to their co-occurring conditions.

Physical Health: Complex ADHD can also have physical health implications. The chronic stress associated with managing ADHD and co-occurring conditions can lead to physical health issues such as sleep disorders, chronic pain conditions, and other stress-related health problems.

In conclusion, Complex ADHD is a multifaceted condition that impacts multiple areas of an individual's life. Understanding these impacts is crucial for developing effective treatment plans and providing appropriate support.

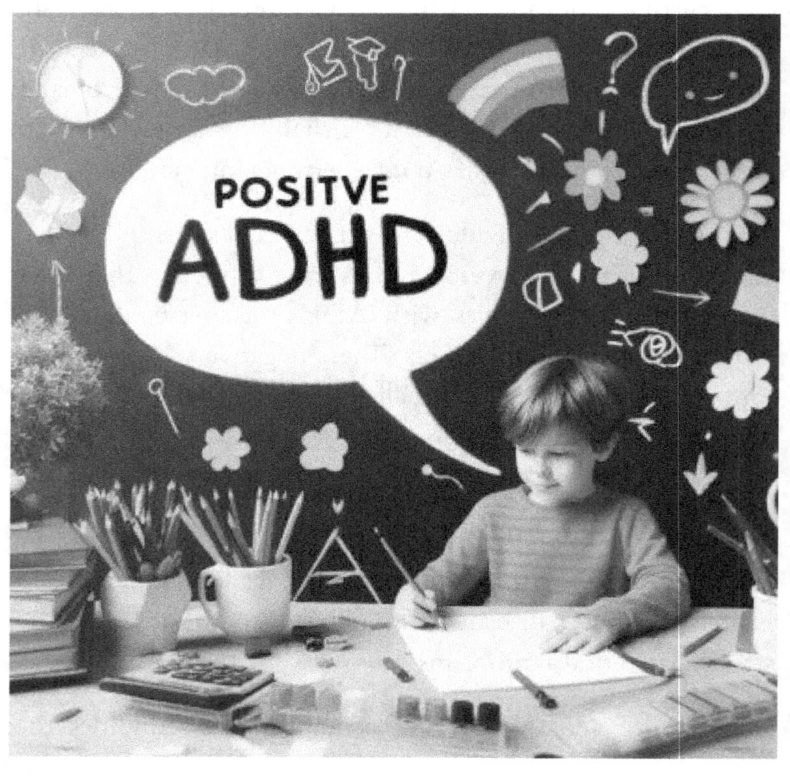
POSITVE
ADHD

Chapter 5: Treatment for Complex ADHD

Therapies used to treat ADHD and Complex ADHD

Therapies used to treat ADHD and Complex PTSD in the UK and Scotland include various psychological and pharmacological interventions. For ADHD, the most common treatments are medication, such as methylphenidate or atomoxetine, and behavioural therapy, such as parent training or cognitive behavioural therapy (CBT).

These treatments aim to reduce the symptoms of inattention, hyperactivity, and impulsivity, and improve the functioning and well-being of people with ADHD. For Complex PTSD, which is a type of PTSD that occurs after repeated or prolonged exposure to trauma, the main treatments are trauma-focused CBT or eye movement desensitisation and reprocessing (EMDR).

These therapies help people process and cope with their traumatic memories, reduce their distress and negative emotions, and enhance their resilience and self-esteem.

In some cases, antidepressants may also be prescribed to help with symptoms of depression or anxiety. In Scotland, there are specific guidelines for delivering evidence-based psychological therapies within NHS Boards, which are summarised in the Matrix document published by NES and the Scottish

Government. The Matrix provides information on the current evidence base, service structures, governance issues and key developmental questions for psychological therapies services.

Medications and other treatments

IN THE **United Kingdom,** the treatment of Attention Deficit Hyperactivity Disorder (ADHD) and Complex Post-Traumatic Stress Disorder (C-PTSD) involves a combination of psychological and pharmacological interventions.

For ADHD, medication is often the first line of treatment. The most commonly prescribed medications include methylphenidate, lisdexamfetamine, dexamfetamine, atomoxetine, and guanfacine1. These medications are not a permanent cure for ADHD but may help someone with the condition concentrate better, be less impulsive, feel calmer, and learn and practise new skills1. Alongside medication, behavioural therapies such as parent training or cognitive behavioural therapy (CBT) are also used to

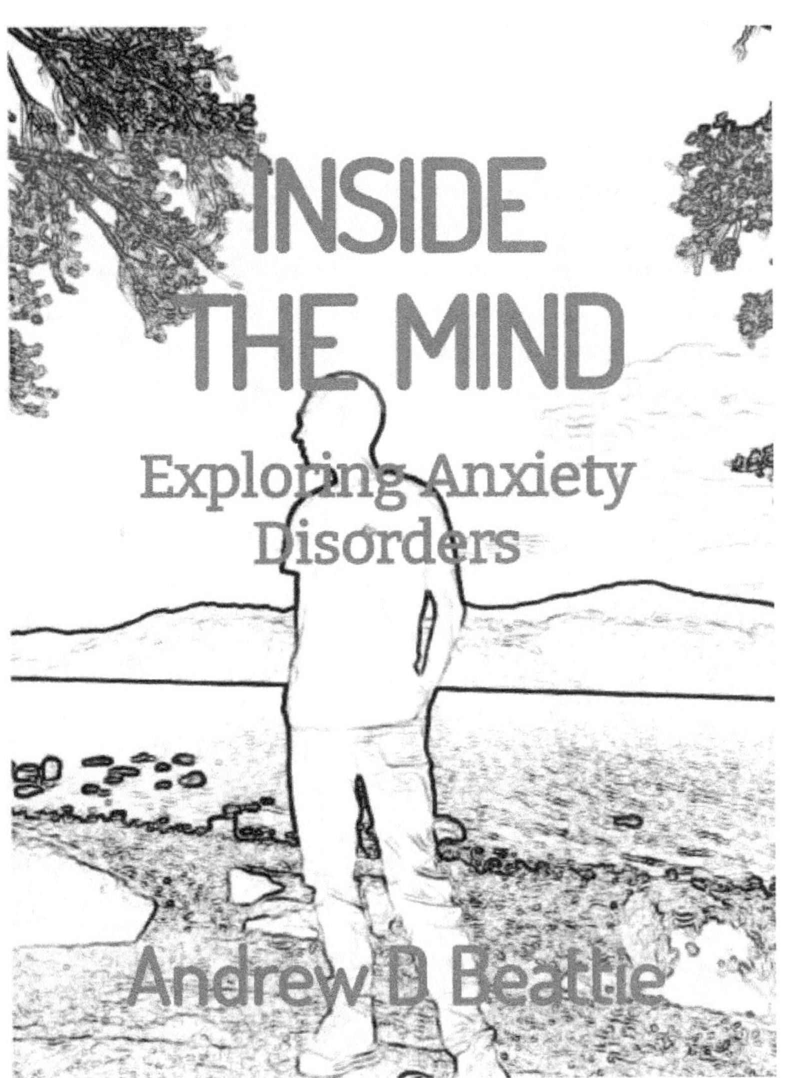
INSIDE
THE MIND
Exploring Anxiety
Disorders
Andrew D Beattie

manage symptoms of ADHD2.

Complex PTSD, a condition that arises after repeated or prolonged exposure to trauma, is primarily treated with trauma-focused therapies. These include trauma-focused cognitive behavioural therapy (CBT) and eye movement desensitisation and reprocessing (EMDR). These therapies aim to help individuals process traumatic memories, reduce distress, and negative emotions, and enhance resilience and self-esteem3. In some cases, antidepressants may also be prescribed to manage symptoms of depression or anxiety associated with C-PTSD

. In **Scotland**, the delivery of these evidence-based psychological therapies within NHS Boards is guided by the Matrix document. This document is published by NES in partnership with the Scottish Government4. It provides a summary of the current evidence base for various therapeutic approaches, guidance on well-functioning psychological therapies services, advice on important governance issues, and key developmental questions for psychological therapies services4. The Matrix document is currently undergoing a comprehensive review process reflecting significant shifts in service delivery and the proliferation of both evidence of effectiveness and demand for psychological therapies and interventions.

Chapter 6: Growing with Complex ADHD

<hr>

How can Complex ADHD impact Children?

Children with complex ADHD face a variety of issues. Here are some of them:

Co-occurring Conditions: Most children and adults with ADHD have one or more co-occurring conditions, which almost always impact treatment and outcomes1. Common conditions co-occurring with ADHD include anxiety, tics, oppositional defiant disorder (ODD), learning disabilities, mood disorders, and substance use disorders.

Impact on Life: ADHD is a chronic, debilitating disorder which may impact upon many aspects of an individual's life, including academic difficulties, social skills problems, and strained parent-child relationships. It can cause disturbances to family and marital functioning.

Persistence into Adulthood: Whereas it was previously thought that children eventually outgrow ADHD, recent studies suggest that 30–60% of affected individuals continue to show significant symptoms of the disorder into adulthood.

Risk of Mental Health Issues: Children with ADHD are more likely than other kids to experience other mental health problems. They're at greater risk for behaviour issues, anxiety, depression, substance abuse, and self-injury3.

Complexity of the Condition: The presence of co-occurring conditions almost always muddles the diagnosis, treatment, and prognosis of ADHD. ADHD and comorbidities may also influence the presentation and severity of one another, which can complicate the detection and treatment of symptoms, and impair overall quality of life

The Teenage Years

COMPLEX ADHD IS A TERM that reflects the common co-occurrence of ADHD with one or more psychiatric, learning, or other neurodevelopmental disorders1. As children with Complex ADHD transition into their teenage years, they may experience a variety of changes and additional symptoms. Here are some potential issues they might face:

Lack of focus: They might have trouble staying on task. They may start a project only to end up starting another before finishing2.

Disorganization: Misplacing items can be a common occurrence. They may spend a lot of time searching for their possessions.

Self-focused behaviour: It can be difficult for them to recognize what other people want or need. They can have a hard time waiting for others or taking turns2.

Fidgeting: Restlessness is a common sign of ADHD. Someone with ADHD might find it difficult to sit still without squirming or getting up2.

Heightened emotionality: Research suggests that people with ADHD may not reach the emotional maturity of a typical 21-year-old until their late 20s or early 30s2.

Fear of rejection: Rejection sensitive dysphoria is common in people with neurodevelopmental disorders such as ADHD. High emotions can be triggered by rejection, teasing, or criticism2.

Daydreaming: A person with ADHD may find themselves lost in daydreams for long periods.

Impulsivity: For a teen with ADHD, resisting temptation may be particularly difficult, potentially leading to dangerous decisions.

It's important to note that the presence of co-occurring conditions almost always muddles the diagnosis, treatment, and prognosis of ADHD. Therefore, recognizing ADHD's "complexity" is of high clinical importance. If you suspect that a teenager is experiencing these symptoms, it's crucial to seek professional help for an accurate diagnosis and appropriate treatment

Transition from Teenager to Adulthood

ADULTS WITH ADHD MAY find they have problems with organisation and time management, following instructions, focusing, and completing tasks, coping with stress, feeling restless or impatient, impulsiveness and risk taking. Some adults may also have issues with relationships or social interaction [2]. The symptoms of ADHD are more difficult to define in adults and tend to be subtler than in children. Generally, adults present less with hyperactivity but exhibit inattentiveness, carelessness, a lack of attention to detail, inability to prioritise and non-completion of tasks, forgetfulness and frequently losing things [3].

ADHD is a neurodevelopmental disorder that is thought to be caused by a combination of genetic and environmental factors. It affects about 5% of children and 2.5% of adults worldwide [4]. In the UK, it is estimated that 3-9% of school-aged children and young people have ADHD [5], but the prevalence of ADHD in adults is not well known. Some studies suggest that about 15% of children with ADHD continue to have a full range of symptoms in adulthood [6].

ADHD can be treated using medication or therapy, or a combination of both. Treatment is usually arranged by a specialist, such as a paediatrician or psychiatrist. Treatment aims to relieve the symptoms and improve the person's functioning and quality of life [1].

Sources:

[1]	https://www.nhsinform.scot/illnesses-and-conditions/mental-health/attention-deficit-hyperactivity-disorder-adhd

[2]	https://www.nhs.uk/conditions/attention-deficit-hyperactivity-disorder-adhd/

[3] https://www.pulsetoday.co.uk/clinical-feature/clinical-areas/mental-health-and-addiction/overdiagnosis-adhd/

[4] https://www.ncbi.nlm.nih.gov/pmc/articles/PMC4195638/

[5] https://www.nice.org.uk/guidance/ng87/chapter/Context

[6] https://www.ncbi.nlm.nih.gov/pmc/articles/PMC1525089/

Supporting a Teenager with Complex ADHD / ADHD

COMPLEX ADHD IS A TERM that describes the frequent coexistence of ADHD with other mental, learning, or neurodevelopmental disorders. Teenagers with Complex ADHD may face various challenges and new symptoms as they grow up. If you know someone who has Complex ADHD, you may wonder how you can help them. Here are some tips:

- Be supportive and understanding. Don't judge them for their difficulties or mistakes. Recognize their strengths and achievements.

- Be patient and flexible. Don't expect them to do things the same way as others. Allow them to work at their own pace and style.

- Be clear and consistent. Give them simple and specific instructions. Remind them of the rules and expectations. Praise them for following them.

- Be organized and structured. Help them create a routine and stick to it. Provide them with reminders and tools to keep track of their tasks and belongings.

- Be encouraging and positive. Help them find activities that interest them and make them happy. Motivate them to pursue their goals and dreams.

It's important to remember that the existence of co-occurring conditions often complicates the diagnosis, treatment, and prognosis of ADHD. Therefore, acknowledging ADHD's "complexity" is very important for clinical practice. If you think that a teenager is showing symptoms of Complex ADHD, it's essential to seek professional help for a precise diagnosis and suitable treatment.

Complex ADHD as an Adult

PEOPLE WITH COMPLEX ADHD may struggle with managing their time, organizing their tasks, staying focused, regulating their emotions, and coping with stress. Navigating life with complex ADHD as an adult can be challenging, but not impossible. Here are some tips that may help:

- Seek professional help. A qualified mental health professional can diagnose complex ADHD and provide treatment options, such as medication, therapy, coaching, or a combination of these. Treatment can help reduce the severity of the symptoms and improve the quality of life.

- Learn about complex ADHD. Educating yourself about the causes, effects, and strategies of complex ADHD can help you understand yourself better and find ways to cope. You can read books, articles, blogs, or podcasts that offer information and advice on complex ADHD. You can also join online or in-person support groups where you can share your experiences and learn from others who have similar challenges.

- Create a routine. Having a consistent daily schedule can help you stay on track and reduce stress. You can use a planner, a calendar, an app, or a reminder system to plan your activities and prioritize your tasks. You can also set alarms or timers to help you manage your time and avoid procrastination.

- Simplify your environment. A cluttered or chaotic environment can make it harder to focus and organize. You can declutter your home, your workspace, and your digital devices by getting rid of unnecessary items, sorting them into categories, and storing them in labelled containers or folders. You can also limit distractions by turning off notifications, wearing headphones, or finding a quiet place to work or study.

- Practice self-care. Living with complex ADHD can be exhausting and stressful. You need to take care of your physical and mental health by getting enough sleep, eating well, exercising regularly, and relaxing. You can also practice mindfulness, meditation, breathing exercises, or other techniques that can help you calm your mind and body.

- Seek support. You don't have to deal with complex ADHD alone. You can reach out to your family, friends, partner, or co-workers who can offer you emotional support, practical help, or feedback. You can also work with a coach, a mentor, or a tutor who can help you develop skills and strategies to overcome your challenges.

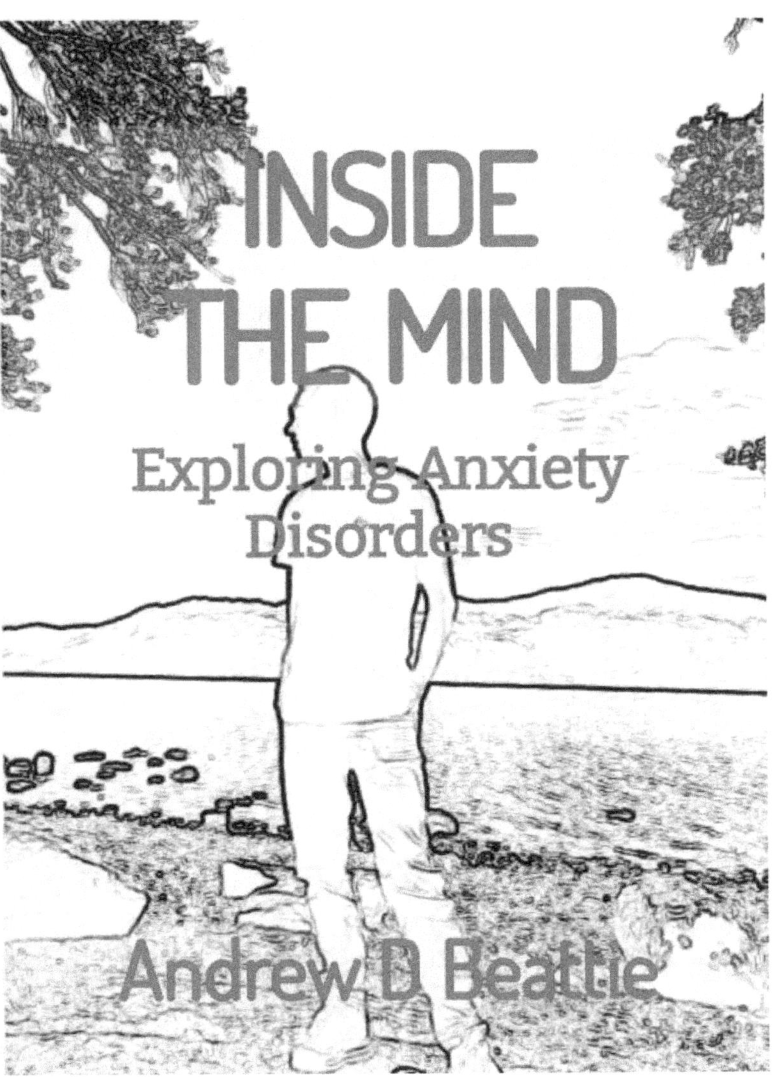
INSIDE
THE MIND
Exploring Anxiety
Disorders
Andrew D Beattie

Chapter 7: Diagnosing Complex ADHD

Complex ADHD is a term that refers to ADHD that co-occurs with one or more other conditions, such as anxiety, learning disabilities, mood disorders, or substance use disorders. These co-existing conditions can make the diagnosis and treatment of ADHD more challenging, as they may influence the presentation and severity of ADHD symptoms and impair the quality of life of individuals with ADHD. Complex ADHD is also influenced by various factors, such as genetics, environment, and neurodevelopmental differences.

According to the NHS, ADHD affects about 2 to 5% of school-aged children and young people in the UK, and about 2% of adults. However, these numbers may vary depending on the diagnostic criteria and methods used. In Scotland, the prevalence of ADHD among children aged 6 to 12 was estimated at 5.8% in 2014, using the Strengths and Difficulties Questionnaire (SDQ).

The treatment of complex ADHD requires a comprehensive approach that considers the needs and preferences of each individual, as well as the impact of co-occurring conditions on their functioning. The treatment options may include medication, psychological therapies, behavioural interventions, educational support, and lifestyle changes. The goal of treatment is to reduce the negative effects of ADHD and co-existing conditions, and to enhance the strengths and abilities of individuals with complex ADHD.

Sources:

- What Is Complex ADHD? Definition, Diagnosis & Treatment - ADDitude (https://www.additudemag.com/complex-adhd-symptoms-diagnosis-treatment/)

- Attention deficit hyperactivity disorder (ADHD) - NHS (https://www.nhs.uk/conditions/attention-deficit-hyperactivity-disorder-adhd/)

- Treatment of Complex ADHD - CHADD (https://chadd.org/continuing-education/treatment-of-complex-adhd/)

- The Difference Between ADD Vs ADHD. Symptoms & Treatments - We Level Up ... (https://welevelupfl.com/behavioral-health/add-vs-adhd/)

- Prevalence of neurodevelopmental disorders among Scottish schoolchildren in 2014: a retrospective cohort study | BMJ Open (https://bmjopen.bmj.com/content/9/7/e028939)

How do you get Diagnosed?

THE PROCESS FOR DIAGNOSIS of Complex ADHD in Scotland, England, Wales, and Northern Ireland may vary depending on the availability of specialists and the waiting time for assessment. However, some general steps are:

- Complex ADHD is a subtype of ADHD that involves co-occurring conditions such as anxiety, depression, bipolar disorder, autism spectrum disorder, or learning difficulties.

- To be diagnosed with Complex ADHD, one must first meet the criteria for ADHD alone, which are based on the DSM-5 or ICD-11 diagnostic manuals.

- The symptoms of ADHD must be present in at least two settings (such as home, school, or work), cause significant impairment in daily functioning, and not be better explained by another condition.

- To get an assessment for ADHD through the NHS, one must first visit a GP and explain why they think they have ADHD. The GP may ask them to fill in a screening tool and then refer them to a specialist for further evaluation.

- The specialist may be a psychiatrist, a paediatrician, an ADHD nurse, or a psychologist. They will conduct a detailed assessment that may involve interviews, questionnaires, observations, and cognitive tests.

- The specialist will also screen for any co-occurring conditions that may complicate the diagnosis and treatment of ADHD. They may use additional tools or criteria to identify these conditions.

- If the specialist confirms the diagnosis of Complex ADHD, they will discuss the treatment options with the patient and their family. These may include medication, psychological therapies, or a combination of both.

The process for diagnosis of Complex ADHD may differ slightly in each country of the UK due to different policies and guidelines. For example:

- **In Scotland**, there is a national clinical guideline for the diagnosis and management of ADHD in children and young people that was published in 2018. It provides recommendations on how to assess and treat ADHD and its co-occurring conditions.

- **In England and Wales**, there is a national institute for health and care excellence (NICE) guideline for the diagnosis and management of ADHD in children, young people and adults that was updated in 2018. It also provides recommendations on how to assess and treat ADHD and its co-occurring conditions.

- **In Northern Ireland**, there is no specific guideline for ADHD, but the health and social care board (HSCB) has issued a service specification for child and adolescent mental health services (CAMHS) that covers the assessment and treatment of ADHD and other mental health conditions.

Therefore, depending on where one lives in the UK, they may encounter different procedures and standards for the diagnosis of Complex ADHD. However, the general principles of assessment and treatment are similar across the UK

.- **US:** The diagnosis of Complex ADHD is based on the DSM-5 criteria for ADHD and the presence of one or more comorbid conditions. The diagnosis should be made by a clinician trained in assessing comorbid conditions, or in consultation with a specialist. The diagnosis should include a comprehensive evaluation of the patient's medical, developmental, educational, and psychosocial history, as well as standardized rating scales, interviews, and observations. The treatment of Complex ADHD should involve a multimodal approach that includes medication, psychosocial interventions, and educational accommodations .

- **Canada:** The diagnosis of Complex ADHD is based on the DSM-5 criteria for ADHD and the presence of one or more comorbid conditions. The diagnosis should be made by a clinician trained in assessing comorbid conditions, or in consultation with a specialist. The diagnosis should include a comprehensive evaluation of the patient's medical, developmental, educational, and psychosocial history, as well as standardized rating scales, interviews, and observations. The treatment of Complex ADHD should involve a multimodal approach that includes medication, psychosocial interventions, and educational accommodations .

- **Australia:** The diagnosis of Complex ADHD is based on the DSM-5 criteria for ADHD and the presence of one or more comorbid conditions. The diagnosis should be made by a psychiatrist trained in assessing comorbid conditions, or in consultation with a specialist. The diagnosis should include a comprehensive evaluation of the patient's medical, developmental, educational, and psychosocial history, as well as standardized rating scales, interviews, and observations. The treatment of Complex ADHD should involve a multimodal approach that includes medication, psychosocial interventions, and educational accommodations .

- **New Zealand:** The diagnosis of Complex ADHD is based on the DSM-5 criteria for ADHD and the presence of one or more comorbid conditions. The diagnosis should be made by a psychiatrist trained in assessing comorbid conditions, or in consultation with a specialist. The diagnosis should include a comprehensive evaluation of the patient's medical, developmental, educational, and psychosocial history, as well as standardized rating scales, interviews, and observations. The treatment of Complex ADHD should involve a multimodal approach that includes medication, psychosocial interventions, and educational accommodations .

:   https://www.additudemag.com/complex-adhd-symptoms-diagnosis-treatment/

:   https://www.ranzcp.org/practice-education/guidelines-and-resources-for-practice/adult-adhd-practice-guidelines

:   https://www.cahs.health.wa.gov.au/Our-services/Mental-Health/Specialist-services-and-day-programs/Complex-Attention-and-Hyperactivity-Disorders-Service

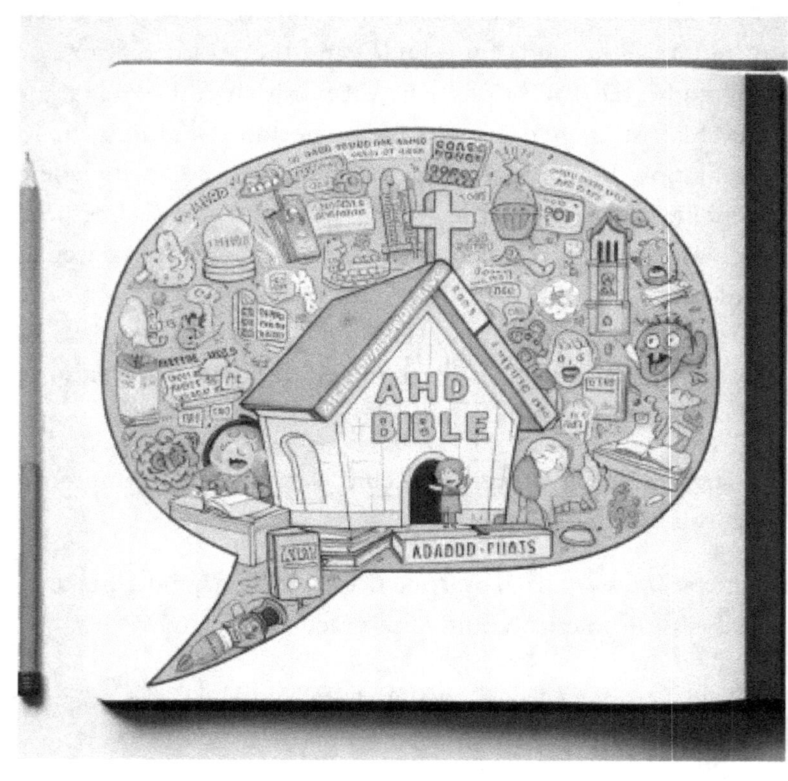

Chapter 8: Self Screening Tools

Self-assessment tools for ADHD can be useful to screen for the condition and to monitor the treatment response, but they are not very accurate by themselves. They have some limitations, such as:

- They are not standardized or validated for different populations, cultures, or settings .

- They rely on self-report, which can be biased by memory, mood, or social desirability.

- They do not capture the developmental history, the functional impairment, or the comorbid conditions that are essential for a proper diagnosis .

Therefore, self-assessment tools for ADHD should always be complemented by a comprehensive clinical evaluation by a qualified and licensed healthcare provider . This evaluation should include:

- A detailed interview with the individual and, if possible, a family member or a close informant

- A review of medical, educational, and psychological records

- A physical examination and laboratory tests to rule out any medical causes of the symptoms

- A neuropsychological assessment to measure cognitive abilities, attention, executive functions, memory, and learning

- A behavioural observation in different settings (e.g., home, school, work)

- A use of standardized rating scales and checklists from multiple sources (e.g., self, parent, teacher, spouse)

If you are wondering if you have adult ADHD, you may want to take an online screening tool to get an indication of whether you might benefit from further clinical evaluation. Online screening tools are not diagnostic tests, but they can help you recognize the signs and symptoms of adult ADHD and decide if you need professional help. There are several online screening tools available, but some of the best ones are:

- **The Adult Self-Report Scale (ASRS) Screener** developed by the World Health Organization and the Workgroup on Adult ADHD. This is a short questionnaire that asks you about six common symptoms of adult ADHD. Scoring four or more on this screener suggests that you may have ADHD and should seek further assessment. You can find this screener online at https://add.org/adhd-test/ or https://adhduk.co.uk/adult-adhd-screening-survey/.

- **The Adult ADHD Clinical Diagnostic Scale (ACDS) v1.2** developed by Dr. Joseph Biederman and colleagues at Massachusetts General Hospital. This is a more comprehensive questionnaire that asks you about 18 symptoms of adult ADHD, as well as your impairment, family history, and comorbid conditions. This scale can help you and your clinician determine if you meet the diagnostic criteria for adult ADHD according to the DSM-IV. You can find this scale online at https://www.aafp.org/family-physician/patient-care/ prevention-wellness/emotional-wellbeing/adhd-toolkit/ assessment-and-diagnosis.html.

- **The Adult ADHD Self-Report Screening Scale for DSM-5 (ASRS DSM-5) Screener** developed by Dr. Lenard Adler and colleagues at New York University School of Medicine. This is a newer version of the ASRS Screener that reflects the updated diagnostic criteria for adult ADHD according to the DSM-5. This screener asks you about nine symptoms of adult ADHD and how often they interfere with your functioning. Scoring six or more on this screener suggests that you may have ADHD and should seek further assessment. You can find this screener online at https://www.aafp.org/family-physician/patient-care/ prevention-wellness/emotional-wellbeing/adhd-toolkit/ assessment-and-diagnosis.html.

These are some of the best online screening tools for adult ADHD, but they are not substitutes for a professional diagnosis. Only a qualified clinician can accurately diagnose adult ADHD and rule out other possible causes of your symptoms. If you score high on any of these screeners, you should consult with your doctor or a mental health professional who specializes in adult ADHD.

ANDREW D BEATTIE

A-Z

Of Mental Health

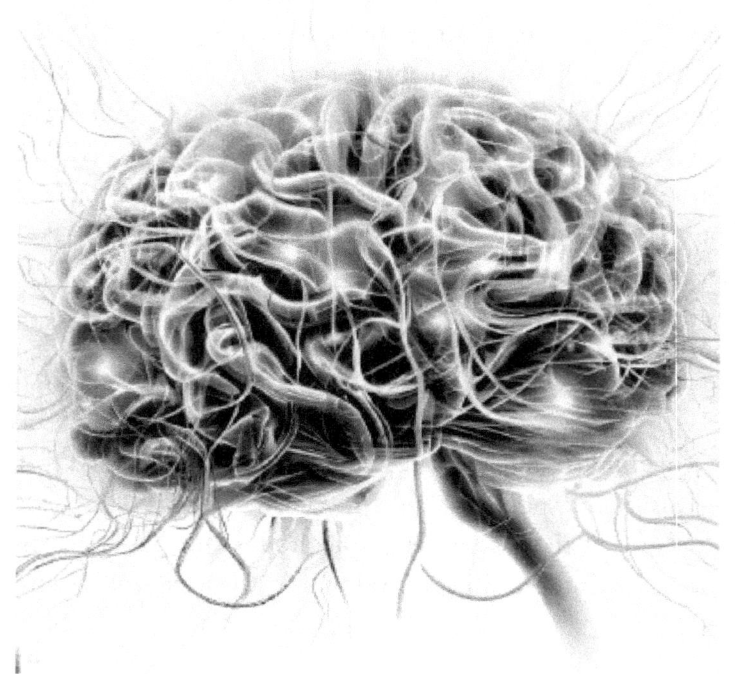

Andrew D Beattie

Chapter 9: What if it isn't Complex ADHD?

Complex ADHD is a term that some people use to describe a combination of ADHD symptoms and other mental health conditions, such as anxiety, depression, bipolar disorder, or PTSD. However, complex ADHD is not an official diagnosis, and it may not accurately capture the underlying causes of the difficulties that people face. Therefore, it is important to seek a comprehensive evaluation from a qualified mental health professional who can assess the full range of possible factors that may contribute to the challenges that people with complex ADHD experience. Some of the alternative explanations that may be considered are:

- **A different type of ADHD:** There are three subtypes of ADHD: predominantly inattentive, predominantly hyperactive-impulsive, and combined. Each subtype has its own set of symptoms and challenges, and some people may switch between subtypes over time. Depending on the subtype, the presentation of ADHD may vary significantly, and some symptoms may be more noticeable or problematic than others.

- **A learning disability or a cognitive impairment:** Some people with ADHD may also have a learning disability or a cognitive impairment that affects their ability to process information, learn new skills, or perform certain tasks. For example, dyslexia can cause difficulty reading, writing, or spelling; dyscalculia can cause difficulty with math; dysgraphia can cause difficulty with handwriting; dyspraxia can cause difficulty with motor skills; or executive function disorder can cause difficulty with planning, organizing, or self-regulating. These difficulties can interfere with academic achievement, work performance, or daily functioning and may require specialized interventions or accommodations.

- A medical condition or a medication side effect: Some medical conditions or medications can mimic or worsen the symptoms of ADHD. For example, thyroid disorders can affect mood, energy levels, or metabolism; sleep disorders can affect attention span, alertness, or mood; iron deficiency can affect cognitive function, memory, or concentration; hormonal changes can affect mood swings, irritability, or impulsivity; or allergies can affect inflammation, brain fog, or fatigue. Some medications can also have side effects that resemble those of ADHD, such as stimulants (e.g., caffeine), antidepressants (e.g., SSRIs), antihistamines (e.g., Benadryl), or steroids (e.g., prednisone). Therefore, it is important to rule out any medical issues or medication interactions that may affect the symptoms of ADHD.

Failure to diagnose ADHD

FAILURE TO DIAGNOSE ADHD can have serious consequences for individuals and society. ADHD is a neurodevelopmental disorder that affects about 5% of children and 3% of adults worldwide. It is characterised by persistent and impairing levels of inattention, hyperactivity and impulsivity that interfere with daily functioning and development. People with ADHD may experience difficulties in various domains of life, such as education, work, relationships, mental health, and physical health.

In the UK, there is a significant gap between the estimated prevalence of ADHD and the actual number of people who receive a diagnosis and treatment. According to a consensus statement by experts and stakeholders, the failure of healthcare provision for ADHD in the UK is due to several factors, such as lack of awareness, stigma, insufficient funding, inadequate training, long waiting times and fragmented services. These barriers prevent many people from accessing timely and appropriate care for their condition, leading to increased risks of poor outcomes and reduced quality of life.

The situation may vary across different regions of the UK, as different health boards have different policies and practices regarding ADHD assessment and treatment. For example, in **Scotland,** there is a pilot project to implement a single diagnostic pathway for ADHD diagnosis in four health boards, which aims to improve the consistency and efficiency of the process. However, there are still challenges and inconsistencies in accessing support for ADHD in Scotland, especially in education. A report by the Scottish ADHD Coalition found that pupils with ADHD are often failed by Scottish schools, due to teachers' lack of knowledge, cuts to school budgets and difficulties in obtaining additional support.

Therefore, it is important to raise awareness and advocate for better provision of services for people with ADHD across the

UK. The Scottish ADHD Coalition has published a guide to adult ADHD assessment, which provides useful information and advice for adults who suspect they may have ADHD and want to seek an assessment. The guide covers topics such as how to prepare for an assessment, what to expect during and after an assessment, how to access treatment and support, and how to cope with common challenges. The guide also includes links to relevant resources and organisations that can help people with ADHD in Scotland.

: Polanczyk G., de Lima M.S., Horta B.L., Biederman J., Rohde L.A. (2007). The worldwide prevalence of ADHD: a systematic review and metaregression analysis. American Journal of Psychiatry 164(6):942-948.

: Young S., Asherson P., Lloyd T., et al. (2021). Failure of Healthcare Provision for Attention-Deficit/Hyperactivity Disorder in the United Kingdom: A Consensus Statement. Frontiers in Psychiatry 12:649399.

: Scottish ADHD Coalition (2018). Pupils with attention deficit hyperactivity disorder (ADHD) are being "failed" by Scottish schools.

: BBC News (2021). Cost of living: 'I have to ration my ADHD medication'.

: Scottish ADHD Coalition (2019). Guide to adult ADHD assessment.

Self-harming Behaviour:

ACCORDING TO SOME SOURCES, people with attention-deficit hyperactivity disorder (ADHD) have a higher risk of suicidal behaviour, especially if they have comorbid psychiatric disorders. However, the exact rates of suicide and self-harm among complex ADHD sufferers in the UK are not easy to find. One report from Public Health England in 2016 estimated that the prevalence of ADHD among children and young people in London was 1.7% but did not provide data on suicidal outcomes. Another report from the Mental Health Foundation in 2019 stated that 20.6% of people in the UK had suicidal thoughts at some point in their lives, and 6.7% had attempted suicide, but did not specify the proportion of those with ADHD. Therefore, to answer the question of what are the instances of suicide and self-harm among complex ADHD sufferers in the UK, more research is needed to collect and analyse data on this specific population. A possible breakdown for each home nation could be based on the regional variations in suicide rates reported by the Office for National Statistics, but this would not account for the differences in ADHD prevalence or complexity.

Scotland:

ACCORDING TO THE SCOTTISH Health Survey 2019, the prevalence of self-harm among 13-15 year olds in Scotland was 13.2%, and the prevalence of suicidal thoughts among 16-24 year olds was 9.6%. However, these figures do not specify the diagnosis of the respondents, and there is limited data on the rates of self-harm and suicide among complex ADHD sufferers in Scotland or the UK.

Complex ADHD is a term used to describe ADHD that is accompanied by other mental health conditions, such as depression, anxiety, bipolar disorder, or substance use disorder. These conditions can increase the risk of self-harm and suicide in people with ADHD .

A 2017 research review found that people with ADHD had a higher risk of suicide than the general population, regardless of age. A 2020 research review found that children and adolescents with ADHD had a higher risk of suicidal behaviour or suicide attempts than their peers without ADHD. Both reviews suggested that other factors, such as gender, education, family environment, and co-occurring mental health conditions, could also influence the suicide risk in people with ADHD.

There is no official data on the breakdown of suicide and self-harm rates for each home nation in the UK among complex ADHD sufferers. However, some sources indicate that Scotland has the highest suicide rate in the UK overall, followed by Wales, Northern Ireland, and England . It is possible that this trend also applies to complex ADHD sufferers, but more research is needed to confirm this.

Chapter 10: The State of Mental Health Care In the UK

The state of mental health services in all 4 countries of the UK is a complex and multifaceted issue. According to the NHS website, there are different types of mental health services available, such as urgent helplines, talking therapies, local charities, and specialised care for different groups of people. However, these services may vary in quality, accessibility and availability depending on the location, funding, and demand.

Some of the challenges facing mental health services in the UK include:

- **The impact of the COVID-19** pandemic on people's mental health and wellbeing, as well as on the capacity and delivery of mental health services.

- **The stigma and discrimination** that still exist around mental health problems, which may prevent some people from seeking help or receiving adequate support.

- **The lack of parity** between physical and mental health care, which means that mental health services are often underfunded, understaffed, and overstretched compared to physical health services.

- **The gaps and inequalities** in mental health provision across different regions, age groups, ethnicities, genders, and socioeconomic backgrounds.

- **The need for more prevention,** early intervention, and community-based care, as well as more integration and collaboration between different sectors and agencies involved in mental health care.

To address these challenges, various initiatives and reforms have been proposed or implemented by the UK government and devolved administrations, such as:

- The NHS Long Term Plan for England, which aims to improve access, quality, and outcomes of mental health care by 2023/24.

- The Mental Health (Wales) Measure 2010, which introduced new legal duties for local health boards and local authorities to provide more comprehensive and coordinated mental health services in Wales.

- The Mental Health Strategy for Scotland 2017-2027, which sets out 40 actions to improve mental health care across Scotland, with a focus on prevention, early intervention, and recovery.

- The Protect Life 2 strategy for Northern Ireland, which outlines a range of measures to reduce suicide and self-harm, as well as to promote positive mental health and resilience in Northern Ireland.

These initiatives and reforms are expected to bring positive changes and improvements to the state of mental health services in all 4 countries of the UK. However, they also require sustained investment, commitment, and evaluation to ensure that they meet the needs and expectations of the people who use them.

References:

: https://www.nhs.uk/nhs-services/mental-health-services/

: https://www.mind.org.uk/news-campaigns/news/mind-reveals-true-extent-of-crisis-in-mental-healthcare-with-more-than-17000-reports-of-serious-incidents-in-past-year-alone/

: https://www.kingsfund.org.uk/projects/positions/mental-health

: https://www.england.nhs.uk/mental-health/about/

: https://gov.wales/mental-health-wales-measure

: https://www.gov.scot/publications/mental-health-strategy-2017-2027/

: https://www.health-ni.gov.uk/publications/protect-life-2-strategy-prevent-suicide-and-self-harm-northern-ireland

Chapter 11: Recovery Stories

—

Emily's Story:

- I was diagnosed with complex ADHD when I was 25 years old. I had always struggled with attention, impulsivity, and emotional regulation, but I didn't know why. I felt like I was constantly failing at everything I tried, and I had low self-esteem and anxiety. I decided to seek help after a major breakdown at work, and that's when I learned that I had complex ADHD. It was a relief to finally have an explanation, but also a challenge to accept and cope with it. I started taking medication and going to therapy, and I learned a lot about myself and how to manage my symptoms. I also joined a support group where I met other people who understood what I was going through. It was not easy, but it was worth it. Today, I have a fulfilling career, a loving partner, and a positive outlook on life. I still have complex ADHD, but it doesn't define me or limit me.

COMPLEX ADHD

Walter's Journey:

- My journey with complex ADHD began when I was a child. I was always restless, hyperactive, and easily distracted. I had trouble following rules and instructions, and I often got into trouble at school and at home. My parents and teachers thought I was lazy, rebellious, and disrespectful. They didn't know that I had complex ADHD, and neither did I. I grew up feeling misunderstood and isolated, and I developed depression and substance abuse problems. It wasn't until I was 32 years old that I finally got diagnosed with complex ADHD. It was a turning point in my life. I realized that I had a neurodevelopmental disorder that affected my brain function, and that it was not my fault. I started taking medication and attending counselling sessions, and I gradually learned how to cope with my complex ADHD. I also found a mentor who helped me discover my strengths and passions. Today, I am a successful entrepreneur, a happy father, and a proud advocate for complex ADHD awareness.

Lucy's Story:

- Complex ADHD has been a part of my life since I can remember. I always had difficulty concentrating, organizing, and planning. I was easily bored, frustrated, and overwhelmed. I had trouble making friends and fitting in. I felt like an outsider who didn't belong anywhere. I didn't know that I had complex ADHD until I was 18 years old, when I went to college and realized that I couldn't keep up with the academic demands. I was failing my classes and losing my motivation. That's when I decided to seek professional help, and that's when I found out that I had complex ADHD. It was a shock, but also a relief. It explained so much about my struggles and challenges. It also gave me hope that things could get better. I started taking medication and participating in cognitive-behavioural therapy, and I noticed a significant improvement in my attention, memory, and mood. I also joined a student organization where I met other people who had complex ADHD or other learning disabilities. They became my friends and my support system. Today, I am a confident college graduate, a passionate teacher, and a hopeful learner.

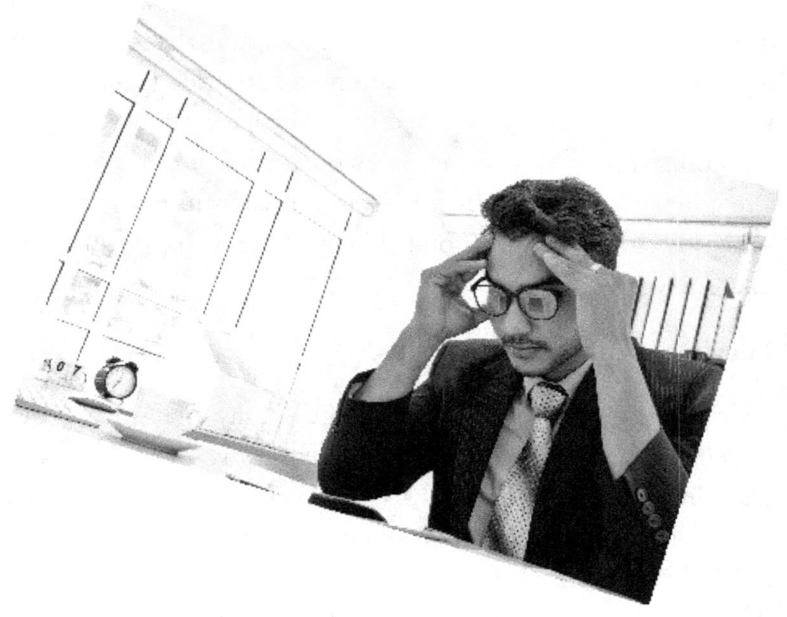

Chapter 12: Support

Attention deficit hyperactivity disorder (ADHD) is a condition that affects the behaviour and attention span of children and adults. People with ADHD may have difficulty concentrating, following instructions, organizing themselves, or controlling their impulses. ADHD can cause problems at home, school, work, and in social situations.

There are various sources of support available to patients and families in the UK who are dealing with ADHD. The NHS provides diagnosis and treatment options, such as medication and therapy, for people with ADHD. The NHS website has more information about the symptoms, causes, and treatments of ADHD.

In addition to the NHS, there are also several voluntary organizations that offer support and information to people with ADHD and their families. Some of these organizations are:

- **Scottish ADHD Coalition** - A national charity that brings together all the ADHD support groups in Scotland. It provides local support, online resources, events, and advocacy for people with ADHD in Scotland.

- **ADDISS** - The Attention Deficit Disorder Information and Support Service is a national charity for ADD/ADHD in the UK. It offers a helpline, training courses, publications, conferences, and a network of local support groups.

- **HACSG** - The Hyperactive Children's Support Group is a national charity that advocates a non-medication approach to ADD/ADHD. It provides dietary advice, newsletters, books, and research updates.

- **UK ADHD Partnership** - A group of professionals who work with children and young people with ADHD. It aims to improve the quality of care and services for people with ADHD in the UK. It also lists some local support groups on its website.

These are some of the sources of support available to patients and families in the UK in dealing with ADHD. For more information, please visit the websites of these organizations or contact them directly.

Conclusion:

You have reached the end of this book, but not the end of your journey. Complex ADHD is a condition that affects many aspects of your life, but it does not define who you are. You have learned about what it is, how it manifests, how it can be diagnosed and treated, and how to cope with its challenges. You have also read some personal stories from people who share your struggles and successes. I hope that this book has given you some insight, inspiration, and encouragement to pursue your goals and dreams.

Complex ADHD is not a curse, but a gift. It gives you a unique perspective, a creative mind, and a passionate heart. You have strengths and talents that can make a positive difference in the world. You are not alone, but part of a community that supports and understands you. You deserve respect, compassion, and happiness. Remember that you are more than your symptoms, and that you can overcome any obstacle with the right mindset and tools.

Thank you for reading this book, and for taking the first step towards a better life. I hope that you will continue to explore, learn, and grow as a person with Complex ADHD. You have the power to create your own story, and to make it a wonderful one. I wish you all the best in your future endeavours

ANDREW D BEATTIE

ALL MY BOOKS ARE AVAILABLE FROM THE FOLLOWING:

Search "AndrewDBeattie"

Or from my website:

www.andrewdbeattie.co.uk[1]

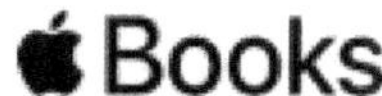

ALL MY BOOKS ARE AVAILABLE FROM THE FOLLOWING:

---

1. http://www.andrewdbeattie.co.uk

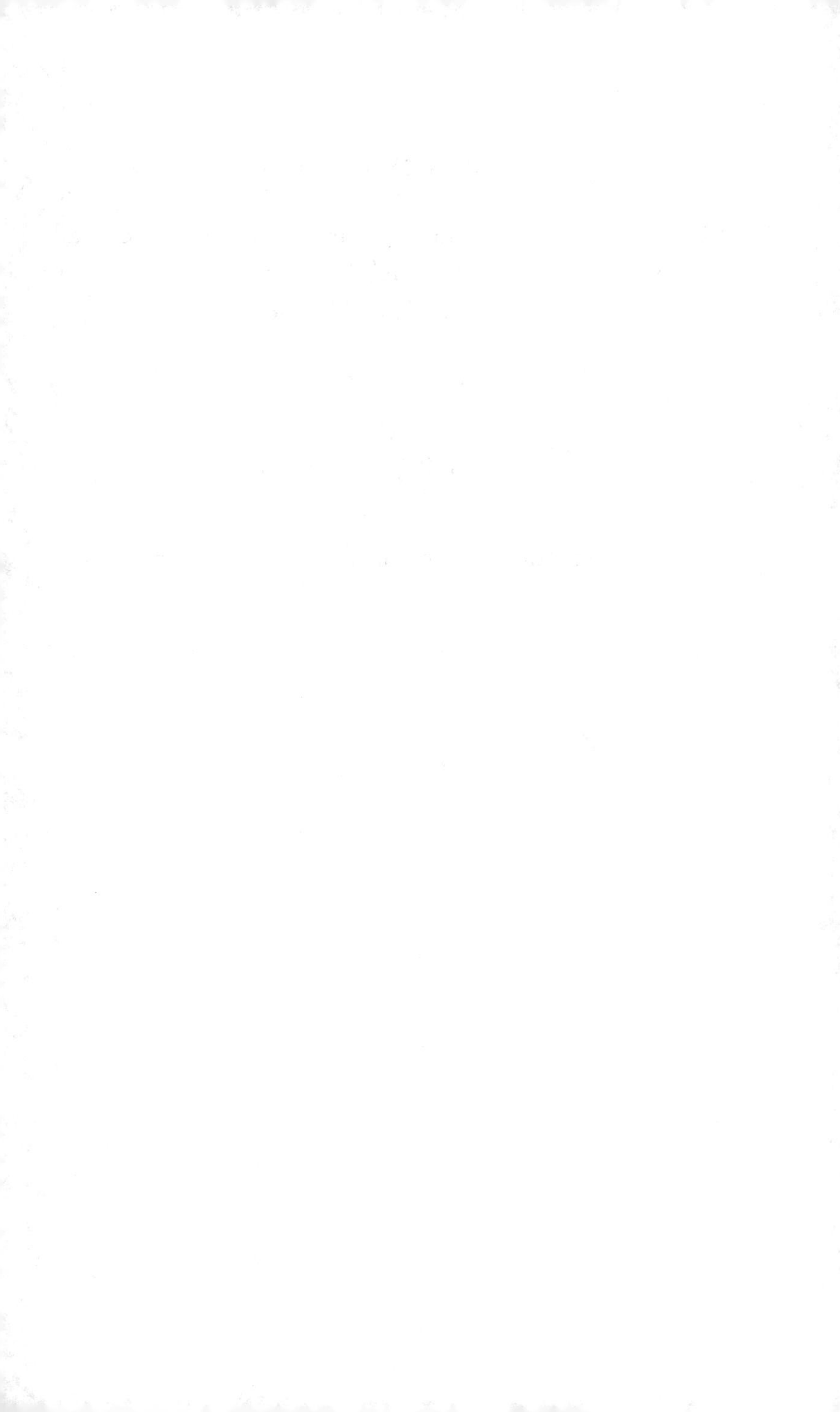

Don't miss out!

Visit the website below and you can sign up to receive emails whenever Andrew D Beattie publishes a new book. There's no charge and no obligation.

https://books2read.com/r/B-A-MYHZ-EQOPC

BOOKS2READ

Connecting independent readers to independent writers.

Did you love *Complex ADHD*? Then you should read *INSIDE THE MIND - Exploring Anxiety Disorders*[2] by Andrew D Beattie!

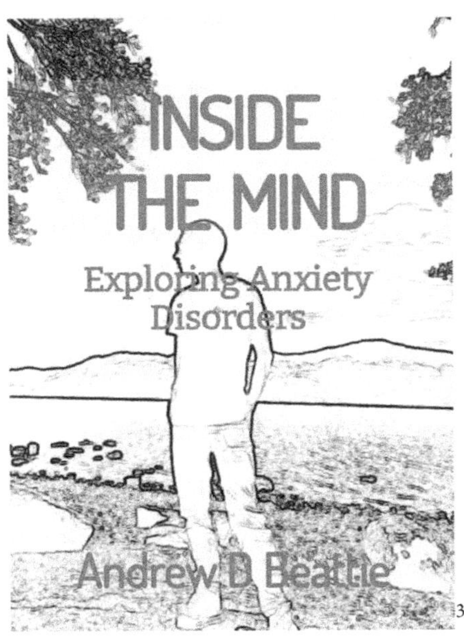

[3]

"INSIDE THE MIND - Exploring Anxiety Disorders" is your essential guide to understanding one of the most common yet misunderstood mental health issues. This book delves deeply into the complexities of anxiety disorders, serving as a valuable resource for sufferers, caregivers, and healthcare professionals alike.

This comprehensive guide covers a wide range of conditions from Generalized Anxiety Disorder to Social Anxiety and Panic

---

2. https://books2read.com/u/3yQgPZ

3. https://books2read.com/u/3yQgPZ

Disorders. Discover their symptoms, causes, and life-altering effects, all presented with real-life case studies and the latest scientific research. But this book doesn't stop at diagnosis; it explores various treatment options including therapy, medication, and lifestyle changes, empowering you to take control of your mental health.

The book also aims to dismantle stigmas and misconceptions surrounding anxiety disorders. Through accessible language and a compassionate tone, the authors initiate an open dialogue, aiming to reduce shame and inspire hope. This approach makes complex medical terminology digestible for readers of all backgrounds, ensuring no one feels isolated in their struggle.

Also by Andrew D Beattie

All About
All About Crohn's Disease

A - Z
A - Z of Mental Health

Inside The Mind
Complex ADHD

Mental Health
Breaking Through Executive Dysfunction: Strategies for
Patients with Complex Trauma and ADHD
Anxiety Disorders Unmasked - Tackling Procrastination Head
On
INSIDE THE MIND - Exploring Anxiety Disorders
Personality Traits Explained

Standalone
My Naked Soul